FRESH START

A GUIDE TO ELIMINATING UNHEALTHY STRESS

SARAH O'FLAHERTY

JOIN MY VIP CLUB

Get Sarah O'Flaherty's first book FOR FREE

Sign up for the no-spam newsletter and
get what other readers have called a great little book full of good
advice, SIMPLIFY YOUR LIFE, for free.

Details can be found at the end of this book.

1

WHAT IS STRESS?

Stress is estimated to cost American businesses up to $300 billion a year and has been labelled the 'health epidemic of the 21st century' by the World Health Organisation [1]. Numerous studies show that job stress is by far the major source of stress for many adults, and in a recent global survey, employers identified stress as the number one health risk factor for their employees [2]. However, stress is not limited to the workplace and can be caused by many things. It can be caused by being stuck in heavy traffic, by having overdue bills, or from having an argument with your neighbour.

It is not surprising then that it is challenging to understand how to manage stress as it has been notoriously difficult to define. Hans Selye, considered to be the father of stress, defined it as the nonspecific response of the body to any demand. Unfortunately, this definition is rather generic and vague. Stress has also been described in a medical sense as the rate of wear and tear on the body, or more broadly, as an aversive event (physical, mental, or emotional) that threatens the well-being of an individual. Other definitions are [3]: the perception of threat with resulting anxiety, discomfort, emotional tension, and difficulty in adjustment; and that stress occurs when environmental demands exceed one's perception of the ability to cope.

However, when considering the many and varied definitions of stress, there was one definition that stood out for me, and that was the three-component definition developed by Kim and Diamond [4]. The authors suggest that this definition can be applied broadly across many settings and situations. First, stress requires heightened excitability or arousal (E). Second, the experience must be perceived as aversive (A). Third, there is a lack of control or uncontrollability (U). Thus, stress can be defined as the product of these three factors and can be shown in the equation outlined below:

$$S = E \times A \times U$$

Having control over an aversive experience is suggested to have a profound mitigating influence on how stressful the experience feels. The *element of control* is the variable that ultimately determines the magnitude of the stress experience and the susceptibility of the individual to suffer the physical and mental impacts of stress.

So, in summary, stress can be defined as a condition in which an individual is aroused by an aversive situation – for example, a hostile employer, or an unpaid bill – with the magnitude of stress and its physiological consequences greatly influenced by the individual's perception of their ability to control the presence or intensity of the situation.

WHAT HAPPENS TO OUR BODIES?

The biological response to stress involves the activation of three major interrelated systems. First, the stressor is perceived by the sensory systems of the brain, which evaluates the stress against how we are now or our current state, and compares it to previous stressful states we have been in. Second, when detecting the stressful challenge, the brain activates the autonomic nervous system which triggers a rapid release of catecholamine, noradrenaline, and adrenaline, often referred to as the fight or flight response. Third, the brain activates the hypothalamic-pituitary-adrenal (HPA) axis. At this stage, adrenal glucocorticoids are released, enhancing an organisms' resistance and adaptation to stress. This biological response is adaptive when it enhances resilience and facilitates the development of coping mechanisms that can protect against future stressors.

However, stress responses occur on a continuum from adaptive to maladaptive, with maladaptive responses leading to a failure in stress-coping and the establishment of greater vulnerability to the negative side effects of stress. Whether stress affects us positively or negatively is influenced by many factors; timing, intensity, duration, predictability, controllability, genetic background, and the life history of the individual.

IS STRESS HARMFUL?

Stress does have a positive side. A certain level of stress may be necessary and can even be enjoyable when it helps you prepare for something or to take action. For example, if you are taking part in a performance, taking an exam, or if you need to get a piece of work completed by a deadline. In these circumstances, the stress response is keeping you alert and focused.

Our physical reactions to stress are determined by our biological history and the way we respond to danger.

As mentioned previously, your danger response is known as

the fight or flight response and when this happens our bodies release the hormones adrenaline and cortisol. It can be helpful to understand the impact these hormones have on your body.

Adrenaline

The release of adrenaline causes rapid changes to your blood flow and increases your heart rate and breathing. This change allows you to get ready to defend yourself (fight) or to run away (flight). You may also notice that you become pale, sweat more, and your mouth might become dry.

Your body responds in this way in reaction to many types of stress, as if it were a physical threat, but in today's world not all perceived threats are physical. For example, you may be having an argument with someone, but your body may react as if you were being attacked by a lion. If the threat is physical, you are being attacked by a lion, you would run away and so you use the effects of the adrenaline appropriately, and once the danger has passed your body will recover. However, if the stress is emotional as an argument generally is, the effects of the adrenaline subside more slowly, and you may go on feeling agitated for a long time. This physical agitation may result in you thinking about the event for longer than you need to, as your body is reminding you of the event until the agitation goes away. If the causes of stress are long-term, you may find that you are always tensed up to deal with them and are never able to relax. This build-up of tension, as you would imagine, can be very bad both for your physical and mental health.

Cortisol

The other form of stress hormone is cortisol, and while it is present in your body all the time, levels tend to increase in response to stress and danger. In the short-term, its effects are positive, to help you deal with an immediate crisis, but long-term stress means that cortisol builds up and creates many stress-related health problems [5].

Short-term positive effects:

- a quick burst of energy
- decreased sensitivity to pain
- increased immunity
- heightened memory

Long-term negative effects:

- imbalances of blood sugar
- increase in abdominal fat storage
- suppressed thyroid activity
- decreased bone density
- decreased muscle mass
- high blood pressure
- lowered immunity
- less able to think clearly

THE IMPACT OF STRESS

Exposure to mild, intense, controllable, or predictable stressors have been linked to adaptive outcomes such as decreases in anxiety or depressive behaviours [6]. However, chronic and unpredictable stress has been proven to impact health, from increasing the length of time needed for injuries to heal, to negatively affect the aging processes, and decreasing immune function.

Stress also impacts on behaviours that support our well-being, such as sleep and exercise. Stress has been shown to negatively affect sleep behaviours. Pre-sleep stress, for example, watching an aversive film, has been shown to increase the numbers of night waking and to distort overall sleep patterns. Even small amounts of negative stress can have a negative impact. When university students were given an intellectually challenging test that resulted in feelings of inferiority, students sleep patterns were heavily affected.

Stress has also been found to impact on physical activity. Observational studies have found a link between increased stress and decreased physical activity. In one experiment, children were placed in a passive reading or a public speaking group. After participating in their respective activities, the children were given the opportunity to exercise. The results showed that the children in the public speaking group were less likely to engage in exercise than the children in the passive reading (less stressful) group.

STRESSFUL LIFE EVENTS

Stressful life events (SLEs), such as a job loss or dealing with a divorce, are strongly predictive of various illnesses including depression. Constance Hammen [7] is the author of the stress generation hypothesis which suggests that the relationship between SLEs and illnesses may also be able to be considered in reverse, for example, where someone with depression may generate these stressful events due to their maladaptive personality patterns or lack of functioning social support. A depressed person may shape their environment, as well as respond to them, and the consequences of their depression and behaviours may serve to generate stressful conditions and events which in turn cause additional symptoms. Therefore, this hypothesis proposes that individuals are not passive victims of stress, but instead actively contribute, however unconsciously, to creating their own environments.

It is important to point out that we all generate life events through our intentional actions (e.g., we choose to move to a new house), or our unintentional actions (e.g., we have a car accident). What the stress generation hypothesis proposes is that depressed individuals generate higher rates of SLE's than non-depressed individuals' due to their maladaptive characteristics, negative thinking patterns, and behaviours.

AM I MORE VULNERABLE?

Stress generation may be a consequence of intrapersonal vulnerabilities (maladaptive personality patterns) and interpersonal vulnerabilities (disrupted social support). It is now suspected that pre-existing personality, cognitive, and interpersonal vulnerabilities may heighten the generation of SLE's which then predict the onset of depression and other mental health issues.

A negative cognitive style is suggested to be one predictive aspect. Negative cognitive styles can also be defined as negative cognitive schemas (i.e., negative core beliefs about the self, world, or future), a negative inferential style (i.e., a tendency to make global, stable attributions about negative events), or rumination (i.e., the tendency to cognitively elaborate on one's distress). A negative cognitive style may lead to the generation of stress through several mechanisms, the main one being the tendency of negative thinking to result in defeatist interpersonal behaviours that erode an individual's support networks, increasing the chance of tension, conflict, and even rejection.

Childhood maltreatment is also likely to set the stage for stress generation. Emotional abuse may be especially predictive of interpersonal stress generation because the content of the abuse (e.g. harsh criticism, name-calling, hostility) supports the child's development of beliefs that they are worthless and a failure. Childhood maltreatment sets up patterns of negative thinking and underlies dysfunctional behaviours, such as excessive reassurance seeking, that disrupt social support and lead to the generation of stress in interpersonal relationships.

SUMMARY

In summary, stress occurs when we are aroused by an aversive situation, with the magnitude of stress and its physiological consequences influenced by the individual's perception of their ability to control the presence or the intensity of the situation. The element of control is an important aspect. When our bodies react to stress, it can be adaptive or maladaptive, depending on factors such as the timing or duration of the stress and our own individual qualities, such as genetic factors. When stress becomes maladaptive it impacts us negatively, both biologically and behaviourally. Individuals with genetic, early environmental, cognitive, personality, and behavioural vulnerabilities generate higher rates of stressful events that are in part dependent on their own behaviour and characteristics than individuals without these vulnerabilities. And while the claim that individuals create their own stress due to their behaviour may sound like 'blaming the victim', it does mean that the individual can make changes to their thoughts and behaviour that may result in a reduction in any stressors they may have been generating.

2

WHAT IS BURNOUT?

I want to talk a little bit about burnout. I'd heard about stress, and I'd also heard a lot of talk about burnout, which left me wondering, what was the difference between these two terms? While both terms are frequently mentioned, they are often used interchangeably, which creates confusion as to what each means.

If you're finding that constant stress has left you feeling disillusioned, helpless, and exhausted, you may be suffering from burnout. When you're burned-out, things look bleak, problems seem impossible to overcome, and it's difficult to muster up the energy to do anything about your situation.

Burnout has been defined as the prolonged response to chronic emotional and interpersonal stressors, often related to a job, and includes the three dimensions of exhaustion, cynicism, and inefficiency [8]. When you are burned-out you will feel overwhelmed, emotionally drained, and unable to meet the demands of daily life. As the stress continues, things can get progressively worse; your physical health is impacted, you lose your motivation, and your ability to function effectively is reduced.

If you are feeling burned-out, it can be difficult to see a way out. You may be in a job where your boss keeps pushing you for more and you don't know how to say no, or you're worried that if you don't do what you're told you will lose your job. Maybe you'd love to leave the job you're in, but you have a mortgage to pay, and you don't feel you can leave your current job until you find a new one. It's so easy to feel totally stuck!

While burnout should be a major concern for both employers and employees as it reduces productivity and negatively impacts interpersonal relationships, it is often the last thing considered in a busy workplace where both parties ending up suffering from and paying for the fallout.

ARE YOU SUFFERING FROM BURNOUT?

If you can relate to any of the following you may be heading towards burnout:

- Feeling exhausted and the fatigue you feel cannot be relieved by sleep
- losing weight
- not sleeping well
- increasingly depressed
- increased errors and bungling
- feelings of hopelessness and loneliness
- resignation and boredom
- working more and more but accomplishing less and less
- becoming sensitive and touchy about feedback
- feeling like nothing you do makes a difference or is appreciated.

Although not a comprehensive list, these points are a good indication of what you should be watching out for.

WHAT IS THE DIFFERENCE BETWEEN STRESS AND BURNOUT?

Burnout may be the result of unrelenting stress, but it isn't the same as too much stress. Stress generally involves excessive pressures that demand too much of you psychologically and physically. Stressed people can still imagine, however, that if they just get everything under control they'll feel better. Burnout, on the other hand, is about feeling empty, devoid of motivation, and being beyond caring. Individuals experiencing burnout often don't see any hope of positive change in their situations. If excessive stress is like drowning in responsibilities, then burnout is about being all dried up.

Stress
  Characterised by over engagement
  Emotions are over reactive
  Produces urgency and hyperactivity
  Exhausts physical energy
  Leads to anxiety disorders
  Causes disintegration
  Primary damage is physical

Burnout
  Characterised by disengagement
  Emotions are dull and blunted
  Produces helplessness and hopelessness
  Leads to paranoia, detachment, and depression
  Causes demoralisation
  Primary damage is emotional

While stress may kill you prematurely, burnout is more likely to make your life seem not worth living. Another important difference between stress and burnout is that while you're usually aware of being under a lot of stress, you don't always notice burnout when it happens. The symptoms of burnout; hopelessness, cynicism, and detachment from others, can take a while to appear. We often need to be told by those close to use, family or friends, that we are starting to show the effects of burnout. And if this is happening to you, then it's important to listen to those people if they are seeing the warning signs that you are not.

CHARACTERISTICS THAT LEAD TO BURNOUT

Several individual factors have been found to be related to burnout. People who show low levels of hardiness (a sense of control over events, openness to change, and involvement in daily activities) tend to be more prone to burnout. Further, burnout is impacted by the extent to which people believe they have power over the events in their lives, like how a sense of control mitigates stress. Burnout is higher among people who have an external locus of control (they blame outside forces for everything) rather than an internal locus of control (they believe they can influence events and their outcomes). Burnout is also related to low self-esteem, as higher self-esteem means greater resiliency. And people who deal with stressful events in a passive, defensive or avoidant way are more likely to suffer from burnout than those individuals who deal with stressful events in a more active and confronting manner.

WHAT CAN I DO?

Read on, as learning more about what you're dealing with is an excellent first step. Often, when we become burned-out and exhausted we give up important things like self-care (looking after ourselves). I've noted a few points relating to self-care below that are worth considering and actioning immediately:

- Exercise
- Eat well
- Get enough sleep
- Connect with others
- Reframe the way you look at work
- Get a pet
- Learn to say no
- Spend time in nature
- Learn to meditate
- Find a way to give - volunteer, donate, help a friend
- Be grateful - notice what you have, what you can be grateful for
- Foster fun
- Stop being a workaholic.

Some people may consider these points as obvious, and they are, however, they are also the very things that are quickly neglected when we get busy and stressed.

SUMMARY

In summary, burnout is different from stress, it is the prolonged response to chronic emotional and interpersonal stressors, often related to a job, and includes the three dimensions of exhaustion, cynicism, and inefficiency. Some factors that indicate you may be suffering from burnout are losing weight, not sleeping well, or feeling depressed. If you have the following characteristics you may be more prone to suffering from burnout; low hardiness, an external locus of control, low self-esteem, and/or an avoidant or passive coping style. It's important to understand what you're dealing with and why you are suffering from burnout. Usually it's at least partly due to a lack of self-care. If you feel you are heading toward burnout or you feel that you are already suffering from burnout, then make sure you talk to someone (get some support), and implement some self-care practices (see the list above) to help get you started on the road to recovery.

3

THE DIFFERENT WAYS WE COPE

In times of stress, coping includes efforts to solve the problem, attempts to manage one's own emotions, and attempts to manage social relationships. The effectiveness of any coping response will depend on the context in which it occurs. Some examples are; the nature of the stressful situation, the personality characteristics of the individual, the responses of involved others, and the social and cultural context in which the coping process occurs.

No individual coping strategy is ideally suited to all kinds of stress therefore *flexibility in coping* is what is important. So, it is helpful to know and understand the different coping styles available to you.

THE TRANSACTIONAL MODEL

According to the transactional model of stress and coping, the experience of stress is a product of both the person and the situation [9]. The degree of stress experienced by an individual will depend on how they evaluate or appraise a situation. Situations perceived as threatening, harmful, or challenging, that tax our available resources for coping are experienced as stressful. However, if a situation is not considered to be taxing one's resources or ability to cope, it may not be experienced as stress at all. For example, if I need to move to a new location because I have a new job in a new city, I may find this extremely stressful. Especially if I already feel overloaded with work, I must manage all the logistics alone, and I'm not sure I'll like this new job or this new location. However, my friend has just landed her dream job in the city of her choice. She is so happy, and she's recruited friends to help her with her packing. My friend is also moving to a new location, but she hasn't found the same situation stressful at all, in fact she's excited by it. This is because of the way she has viewed it and her strong social support.

The resources one can bring to a stressful situation include one's personality, age, financial assets, education, previous experiences, social support, and physical and mental health. An individual will combine their available resources and their appraisal of the situation to determine which coping response to employ. The coping response may then either be successful or unsuccessful for the individual in assisting to manage their stress.

Coping is a dynamic process that includes efforts to solve the problem (problem-focused), manage emotions (emotion-focused), and maintain close relationships (relationship-focused). People who cope well tend to vary their coping strategies during different phases of a stressor [10]. For example, the initial coping response of someone receiving a diagnosis of cancer may be denial, allowing the person to gradually adapt to the life-threatening disease. However, this may change as the individual and his or her family accept the diagnosis and begin to look toward treatment options. So, although denial is effective initially, if continued it may hinder chances of recovery if treatment isn't sought. Additionally, it is important to be aware that stressful situations may include many different stressors, and these may require different coping responses.

PROBLEM-FOCUSED COPING

Problem-focused coping describes direct efforts to solve the problem at hand. Problem-focused strategies often include trying to change the situation. These strategies may include defining the problem, identifying or generating alternative solutions, coming up with a plan, and then acting on that plan. Other problem-focused coping strategies may be geared toward changing ourselves, such as learning new skills, thereby increasing one's coping resources.

Several factors influence the use of problem-focused coping strategies. For example, the perception of threat or high levels of stress may interfere with the successful use of this form of strategy due to the reduction in capacity for information processing. People are more likely to use problem-focused coping strategies when they feel the situation can be changed and that this change is within their control. For stressful situations that cannot be solved with problem-focused coping such as the death of a family member, individuals may need to direct their efforts to emotion-focused coping.

EMOTION-FOCUSED COPING

The primary focus of emotion-focused coping is to reduce emotional distress. This form of coping may be achieved through avoidance, distance, or wishful thinking. While these strategies can be maladaptive in certain circumstances, they can also be quite effective, as discussed in the cancer example earlier. Changing the meaning of a situation, using cognitive reappraisal, can be helpful when we can't change the problem itself.

RELATIONSHIP-FOCUSED COPING

Relationship-focused coping is aimed at managing, regulating, or preserving relationships during stressful periods. Successful coping may not only involve solving problems and managing emotions, but may also involve maintaining and protecting social relationships, particularly when stressors occur in interpersonal contexts.

This aspect of coping is important for the maintenance of social relationships during periods of stress. In studies of couples coping with stress, relationship-focused coping strategies involving empathic responding have been associated with less marital tension and greater marital satisfaction and stability.

COMBINED COPING

Some coping strategies can have mixed functions. For example, social support seeking could be used to express emotion (emotion-focused coping), to gather information (problem-focused coping), and to maintain relationships with others (relationship-focused coping). Sometimes using a combination of all these strategies together provides an optimal solution for beating stress.

COPING EFFECTIVENESS

While, identifying one ideal coping response would be nice, there is no one strategy that is universally useful for all people across all situations. The effectiveness of a coping strategy depends on; the context in which it occurs (what are the features of the stressful situation), personality factors (what are the features of the person), and social context (who are you interacting with or who is involved in the stressful situation).

Social support has been found to be extremely helpful when dealing with stressful situations. The effect of social support on stress depends on the context of the relationship (e.g., partner, friends, doctor) and the quality of that relationship. Cultural contexts also impact on the effectiveness of coping strategies. For example, the way that individuals seek social support has been found to differ across cultures.

SUMMARY

Two people may use identical coping strategies with different degrees of success, depending on how skilfully the strategy is implemented and their perception of how stressful the situation is. So, while there is no single way of coping, research suggests that successful coping involves resolving the problem, managing emotions associated with the situation, and efforts to manage relationships with others. The ability to be flexible and adapt the coping response to the context in which it occurs appears to be especially useful.

4

OPTIMISM/PESSIMISM AND STRESS

There is a difference in the way that people approach experiences, challenges, and stressors. Those people who are more optimistic in their outlook will tend to expect more positive than negative things to happen to them, whereas people who are more pessimistic in their views tend to expect more negative outcomes. While there are positives and negatives to both perspectives, there is a large body of research that has shown that optimists, when compared to pessimists, adjust better to difficulties. More specifically, optimists tend to adjust better to stress and exposure to a stressor than pessimists. Optimists have been found to experience less psychological distress and less negative impact on their long-term physical well-being.

Stress and the consequences of stress may arise from how people appraise experiences rather than from the experiences themselves. Optimists tend to have a generalized positive outlook about the future, and this impacts how they appraise and approach stressors. Optimists generally report experiencing less distress during stressor exposure compared to pessimists, and it seems that optimism may have a protective role during exposure to a stressor in that optimism acts as a buffer against the adverse impact of stressful events. To understand the underlying components of why optimists deal with stress better, we will look at their goal engagement and choice of coping strategies.

SELF-FULFILLING PROPHESIES

There are often two options when encountering challenges; *engage* to overcome the challenge and achieve goals, or *disengage* to avoid the challenge and give up on the goal. The choice between these two options may depend on whether the desired outcome is perceived to be attainable. Because optimists see positive outcomes as attainable, they are more likely to engage and continue to invest effort to achieve their desired outcome, rather than give-up or disengage as pessimists tend to do.

Several studies have shown how dispositional optimists persist longer on tasks compared with pessimists, in some cases particularly when self-awareness is high, as awareness tends to highlight one's own goals. The tendency for optimists to expect positive outcomes and remain engaged in challenges creates a self-fulfilling prophecy because positive outcomes and success have a greater chance of becoming actualized. On the other hand, for pessimists, the tendency to expect negative outcomes and give up on challenges creates a self-fulfilling prophecy of failure.

COPING

We discussed coping earlier in the book, but as a reminder, coping is central to how people seek to manage internal or external demands. It's about making choices on which coping strategy to use to deal with different types of stress. The main strategies discussed so far have been problem-focused, emotion-focused, relational focused, combined, and approach versus avoidance.

Optimists are more likely to appraise goals as achievable and are more likely to approach challenges and work hard to achieve their goals. Pessimists tend to take the other perspective, they are likely to appraise goals as unachievable, and so are more likely to avoid or disengage from demanding challenges and give up. Optimists are more likely to use a problem-focused strategy or approach strategy.

Research studies have found that optimists are quite flexible in their choice of coping strategy, and will adjust based on the stressor they are dealing with. So, rather than always choosing approach problem-focused coping, optimists will choose approach problem-focused coping when the stressors are controllable, and approach emotional-focused coping when the stressors are less controllable.

MENTAL AND PHYSICAL WELL-BEING

Optimism has consistently been associated with higher levels of psychological well-being, while pessimism has been associated with lower levels of psychological well-being. Optimists have been shown to have better mood and emotional adjustment, better life satisfaction and social support, and are less likely to experience mental health problems, particularly in relation to exposure to stressors. For example, optimists in their first year of college described experiencing less stress, depression, and loneliness as well as feeling more socially supported than their pessimistic colleagues. Because of the large body of research in this area, it can be said that optimism plays a buffering role in the stress-distress relationship.

Optimism has also been linked to better physiological well-being. For example, it has been associated with better physiological well-being in terms of cardiovascular and immune functioning. Compared to pessimists, optimists have also been shown to report less pain, better physical functioning, and to experience fewer physical symptoms. Optimism has also been found to be a significant predictor of good physical health.

It's starting to sound like you need to be an optimist to get by in this world however there is also some contradictory evidence to be found relating to optimists. Several studies have found that optimists, in combination with high-challenge, correlate to lower cellular immunity. One study, exposing participants to a stressful mental effort task, found that optimists displayed goal engagement, and persisted longer than pessimists on the tasks, but also experienced short-term physiological costs. There are also indications that the positive connection between dispositional optimists and goal engagement may involve a higher likelihood of goal conflict, which has been linked to physiological cost through lower immunity.

These results indicate that the engagement displayed by optimists in the face of stressors may be taxing and that although goal engagement may be beneficial in the long run, in the short term there may be physiological costs. However, despite potential short-term costs, the persistence demonstrated by dispositional optimists is likely to be beneficial in the long run, resulting in goal achievement and related to positive physical and psychological well-being.

HOW TO IMPROVE OPTIMISM

There are many positive links between optimism and goal engagement, coping, adjustment, and well-being. Therefore, establishing ways in which optimism can be increased would be beneficial. However, as a personality trait, optimism has been found to be relatively stable. Further, optimism is estimated to be

25% heritable, and financial security, warmth, and attention from parents in childhood may also predict adult-degree of optimism [11].

However, if you don't think you're an optimist, don't panic. I'd say that I tend to be more of a pessimist than an optimist, but we can all work on developing our sense of optimism. One way I've worked to reprogram my brain to have a more positive outlook has been to complete a gratitude journal daily. I make sure that I record at least three positive things, or three things that I am grateful for from each day. Another way this can be achieved is through cognitive behaviour therapies, a therapeutic approach to brain re-training. And it is not a matter of pushing people to 'pull themselves together and become more optimistic', but rather giving people the knowledge and tools to better cope with specific challenges. The development of coping skills contributes to a better outlook, and subsequently a better approach in how to cope with stress.

SUMMARY

Optimism does play a role in how people respond to stressful situations. Optimists tend to expect more good things to happen to them than bad, and when exposed to stressors, they believe in positive outcomes, persist at goal engagement, and use approach coping strategies to deal with the stress at hand. The overall outcome for optimists appears to be better psychological and physiological well-being, including less distress, better life satisfaction, and social support, as well as better cardiovascular and immune functioning. The key questions for you are; how optimistic are you? And are you willing to work on persisting at goal engagement and using approach coping strategies to deal with your life stressors?

5

HOW DO I DEAL WITH STRESS?

The most reported behaviours used to cope with stress include watching TV, surfing the Internet, napping, eating, drinking alcohol, and smoking. Do you use any of these methods to deal with stress? If yes, it's time to look at some other, healthier, more effective options.

Stress management techniques are numerous and include relaxation (e.g., diaphragmatic breathing, guided relaxation), behavioural approaches (e.g., distraction, time management), or cognitive strategies (e.g., humour, positive self-statements). I'll list some starter ideas for you below. Try out a few of these options and then identify which technique you feel would be the most effective for you that you would most likely use. The chosen technique should then be practiced before the stressful event occurs – so you're ready to use it without thinking when a stressful moment arises. Sometimes it can be helpful to set a time each day to practice these techniques. Consider developing mastery with one chosen technique to start with so that it is most likely to be effective when a stressor occurs.

RELAXATION

Relaxation is a voluntary letting go of tension. This tension can be physical tension in the muscles or it can be psychological tension. You may have noticed when you become stressed that you sometimes get a tight feeling in your stomach or you may have trouble breathing. We want to relieve those feelings, and this is where relaxation can help.

When we physically relax, the impulses arising in the various nerves in the muscles change the nature of the signals that are sent to the brain. This change brings about a general feeling of calm, both physically and mentally. Muscle relaxation has a widespread effect on the nervous system and therefore should be a physical treatment, as well as a psychological one.

Muscles are designed to remain in a relaxed state until required to perform some physical activity. Under normal circumstances, a person would show fluctuating patterns of tension and relaxation over the course of the day. However, when the fight or flight response is activated, this creates muscle tension. Unfortunately, these days with so many stressors to deal with, people sometimes allow themselves to be under stress for long periods of time. They seem to forget to turn their fight or flight button off, and so excessive muscle tension becomes constant. Eventually, these people become unable to relax or may not even recognise tension. Because of the constant tension, these individuals may feel jumpy, irritable, tired or apprehensive, or experience frequent headaches and muscle pain.

A continual state of tension makes it easier for a panic attack to occur because the nervous system is already highly aroused. In this case, some minor event, such as getting stuck on a bus for longer than expected, can trigger further tension that can lead to hyperventilation and panic. Even if you do not have panic attacks, you are more likely to feel anxious, constantly apprehensive, or have unpleasant obsessive worries when your body is in a continual state of tension.

Some tension can be good for you, so it is important to learn to discriminate when tension is useful and when it is unnecessary. However, much everyday tension is unnecessary. Only a few muscles are involved in maintaining normal posture, for example, sitting, standing, and walking. Occasionally, an increase in tension is extremely beneficial. For example, it is usually helpful to tense up when you are about to receive a serve in a tennis game. Likewise, it is helpful to tense up and become more alert before a job interview. This tension helps you perform at your best. Do not become frightened of this type of tension.

Tension is unnecessary; when it performs no useful alerting function, when it is too high for the activity involved, or when it remains high after the activating situation has passed. To be more in control of your anxiety, emotions, and general physical well-being, it is important to learn to relax. To do this you need to:

• Learn to recognise tension
• Learn to relax your body
• Learn to let tension go in specific muscles

To recognize tension more readily you should become aware of where in your body you tend to experience tension and the characteristics of this tension – for example, pain, soreness, weakness, or tiredness of muscles. Note also which events in your life or within yourself tend to result in an increase in tension.

CONTROLLED BREATHING

Your degree of body tension is affected by the way you breathe. When you are under stress, you breathe in a fast and shallow way. You can learn to calm yourself by practising controlled breathing exercises. Controlled breathing increases the oxygen flow to the brain, which increases your capacity to think and concentrate.

The following exercises will be useful to you not only in dealing with triggers, but in other efforts and in any life circumstance in which you want or need to calm yourself. Two forms of controlled breathing exercises are offered here: abdominal breathing and calm breathing. Try to practice at least one of these techniques regularly. Five minutes a day for two weeks is a good start. Once you've become comfortable with the techniques, you can use them to combat stress, anxiety, and other stress symptoms.

Abdominal Breathing Exercise

1. Note the level of tension you are feeling. Then place one hand on your abdomen, right beneath your rib cage.

2. Inhale slowly through your nose into the 'bottom' of your lungs – in other words, send the air as low down as you can. When you're breathing from your abdomen, your hand should rise. Your chest should move only slightly while your abdomen expands. In abdominal breathing, the diaphragm – the muscle that separates the lung cavity from the abdominal cavity – moves downward, causing the muscles surrounding the abdominal cavity to push outward.

3. When you've taken a full breath, pause for a moment, and then exhale slowly through your nose or mouth. Be sure to exhale fully. As you exhale, allow your whole body to just let go. You might visualise your arms and legs going limp and loose like a rag doll.

4. Do ten slow, full, abdominal breaths. Try to keep your breathing smooth and regular, without gulping in a big breath or letting your breath out all at once. Remember to pause briefly at the end of each inhalation. Count to ten, progressing with each exhalation. The process should go like this:

Slow inhale ... Pause ... Slow exhale (count 1)
Slow inhale ... Pause ... Slow exhale (count 2)

Slow inhale ... Pause ... Slow exhale (count 3)

and so on up to ten. If you start to feel light-headed while practising abdominal breathing, stop for thirty seconds or so then start up again.

5. Extend the exercise if you wish by doing two or three sets of abdominal breaths, remembering to count to ten for each set (each exhalation counts as one number). Five full minutes of abdominal breathing will have a pronounced effect in reducing anxiety or the early symptoms of panic. Some people prefer to count backwards from ten down to one on each breath. Feel free to do this if you prefer.

Calm Breathing Exercise

1. Breathing from your abdomen, inhale slowly to a count of five (count slowly "1 ... 2 ... 3 ... 4 ... 5" as you inhale).

2. Pause and hold your breath for a count of five.

3. Exhale slowly, through your nose or mouth, to a count of five (or more if it takes you longer). Be sure to exhale fully.

4. When you've exhaled completely, take two breaths in your normal rhythm, then repeat steps one through three in the cycle above.

5. Keep up the exercise for at least five minutes. This should involve going through at least ten cycles of in–five, hold–five, out–five. Remember to take two normal breaths between each cycle. If you start to feel light-headed while practising this exercise, stop for thirty seconds and then start again.

6. Throughout the exercise, keep your breathing smooth and regular, without gulping in breaths or breathing out suddenly.

7. Optional: Each time you exhale, you may wish to say "relax", "calm", "let go", or any other relaxing word or phrase silently to yourself. Allow your whole body to let go as you do this.

PROGRESSIVE MUSCLE RELAXATION

Progressive Muscle Relaxation (PMR) is a systematic technique for achieving a deep state of relaxation. It was developed by Dr. Edmund Jacobson who discovered that a muscle could be relaxed by first tensing it for a few seconds and then releasing it. Tensing and releasing various muscle groups throughout the body produces a deep state of relaxation, which when practiced regularly has been found to reduce physiological symptoms of stress, such as high blood pressure.

PMR is especially helpful for people whose anxiety is strongly associated with muscle tension. Some people experience this as tightness in their neck and shoulders, headaches, backaches, clenching of the jaw, or tenderness around the eyes. Systematically relaxing your muscles can help ease these symptoms of anxiety, as well as help you quiet your mind and manage troubled or racing thoughts. Dr. Jacobson himself once said, "An anxious mind cannot exist in a relaxed body."

A good guideline is to practice PMR for at least twenty minutes per day. Over time, the relaxation experience that you achieve during PMR will generalize to the rest of your day. The regular practice of PMR can go a long way towards helping you to better manage your anxiety, feel more energized, and help you face stressful situations.

The following guidelines are helpful to keep in mind before you begin PMR:

- Find a quiet location to practice where you won't be distracted. Turn off the phone and use a fan or air conditioner to help block out background noise.
- Practice PMR at regular times. Some people choose to use this technique before going to bed, or in the mornings.
- If possible, practice on an empty stomach, as food

digestion after meals can tend to disrupt deep relaxation.

- Get into a comfortable position. Your entire body, including your head, should be supported. Lying down on a sofa or bed or sitting in a reclining chair are two ways of supporting your body most completely. (If you feel sleepy, it is preferable to sit up rather than lay down.)
- Decide not to worry about anything. Give yourself permission to put aside the concerns of the day. Allow taking care of yourself to have precedence over any of your worries.
- Be gentle with yourself – don't judge your performance or worry too much about how well you are practicing the technique. Try to 'let yourself go' and not try to control your body.

Progressive Muscle Relaxation Technique

When you tense a muscle group, do so vigorously, without straining, for 7–10 seconds. Concentrate on what is happening. Feel the build-up of tension in each muscle group. It is often helpful to visualize the muscle group being tensed.

When you release the muscles, do so abruptly, and then relax, enjoying the sudden feeling of limpness. Allow the relaxation to develop for at least 15–20 seconds before going on to the next group of muscles.

Allow all the other muscles in your body to remain relaxed, as far as possible, while working on one group. Tense and relax each muscle group at once. But if an area feels especially tight, you can tense and relax it two or three times.

1. To begin, take three deep abdominal breaths, exhaling slowly each time. As you exhale, imagine that tension throughout your body begins to flow away.

2. Clench your fists. Hold for 7–10 seconds and then release

for 15–20 seconds. Use these same time intervals for all other muscle groups.

3. Tighten your biceps by drawing your forearms up towards your shoulders and 'making a muscle' with both arms. Hold ... and then relax.

4. Tighten your triceps – the muscle on the undersides of your upper arms – by extending your arms out straight and locking your elbows. Hold ... and then relax.

5. Tense the muscles in your forehead by raising your eyebrows as far as you can. Hold ... and then relax. Imagine your forehead muscles becoming smooth and limp as they relax.

6. Tense the muscles around your eyes by clenching your eyelids tightly shut. Hold ... and then relax. Imagine sensations of deep relaxation spreading all around the area of your eyes.

7. Tighten your jaw by opening your mouth so widely that you stretch the muscles around your jaw. Hold ... and then relax. Let your lips part and allow your jaw to hang loose.

8. Tighten the muscles in the back of your neck by pulling your head way back; as if you were going to touch your head to your back (be gentle with this muscle group to avoid injury). Focus only on tensing the muscles in your neck. Hold ... and then relax. Since this area is often especially tight, it's good to do the same tense–relax cycle twice.

9. Take a few deep breaths and tune into the weight of your head sinking into whatever surface it is resting on.

10. Tighten your shoulders by raising them up as if you were going to touch your ears. Hold ... and then relax.

11. Tighten the muscles around your shoulder blades by pushing your shoulder blades back as if you were going to touch them together. Hold the tension in your shoulder blades ... and then relax. Since this area is often especially tense, you might repeat the tense–relax sequence twice.

12. Tighten the muscles of your chest by taking in a deep breath. Hold for up to ten seconds ... and then release slowly.

Imagine any excess tension in your chest flowing away with the exhalation.

13. Tighten your stomach muscles by sucking your stomach in. Hold ... and then release. Imagine a wave of relaxation spreading through your abdomen.

14. Tighten your lower back by arching it up. Hold ... and then relax.

15. Tighten your buttocks by pulling them together. Hold ... and then relax. Imagine the muscles in your hips going loose and limp.

16. Squeeze the muscles in your thighs all the way down to your knees. You will probably have to tighten your hips along with your thighs since the thigh muscles attach at the pelvis. Hold ... and then relax. Feel your thigh muscles smoothing out and relaxing completely.

17. Tighten your calf muscles by pulling your toes toward you (flex carefully to avoid cramps). Hold ... and then relax.

18. Tighten your feet by curling your toes downward. Hold ... and then relax.

19. Mentally scan your body for any residual tension. If a specific area remains tense, repeat one or two tense–relax cycles for that group of muscles.

20. Now imagine a wave of relaxation slowly spreading throughout your body, starting at your head and gradually penetrating every muscle group, all the way down to your toes.

BARRIERS TO RELAXATION

Some people say that they cannot relax, or that they can't bring themselves to practice relaxation. Since all human beings share the same biological make-up there is no reason why relaxation should work for some and not others. The only reason relaxation may not work for some people is usually due to some psychological factor or insufficient practice. These problems can be overcome. Some examples of difficulties are given below.

I am too tense to relax. It is because you are so tense that you need to practice relaxing. And while relaxation may take longer than expected, if you keep working on it you will see the results eventually. Consider if there is another reason why you may not be willing or able to work on relaxing.

I don't like the feelings of relaxation. Some people are so unused to relaxing that when they do finally feel a little relaxed it feels uncomfortable to start with. It is important to remember that it is not healthy for your body to be tense and stressed all the time. Being relaxed is a healthy and normal way for your body to be, you just need to get used to this new feeling.

I feel guilty doing the relaxation exercises. It feels like I'm wasting my time. Again, you need to consider how important it is to get your body back to equilibrium and in a more relaxed state. If you keep allowing yourself to be tense and stressed much of the time, you will be heading toward burnout and it will take even more time and effort to recover from that.

I can't find a place to do my relaxation exercises. If you try hard enough, you will find somewhere. It is a great idea to make your relaxation a bit of a routine, so the same time each day and the same place can be useful. If you're struggling to find a quiet place at home, consider a park or quiet space outdoors.

I don't feel like I'm getting anything out of this. Don't expect relaxation to be an immediate cure-all. It will take some time to have an effect. Remember, that you've likely spent years building up stress and tension. It will not evaporate with one or two relaxation exercises. Give it some time.

Relaxation and breathing exercises are great places to start, however, there are other ways to deal with stress.

ACKNOWLEDGE YOUR PROBLEMS

Sometimes, people let their lives slip into chaos to cover up underlying problems they are not willing to face or are unable to deal with. The only person who can decide if this is happening is you and if you do think that this might describe you, it may be a good idea to consider talking things through with a professional. Why not see a psychologist or a counsellor? Once you've begun to tackle your problems, you will start to feel better and you will be more able to relax.

SLEEP

Sleep is very important to health, and sleep problems, such as insomnia, are a common sign of stress. Lying awake worrying about things can make everything seem a lot worse – and it's late at night or in the small hours of the morning that are the worst times to be focused on your worries. If you find you can't stop worrying, it may help to write a list of the things that are bothering you, or write yourself a letter about them. Once they are recorded, you may be able to switch off and relax more easily. Some people find it very helpful to keep a diary or a journal. You could even think about having a worry journal, a place where you can keep your worries so you know they're safely listed. You can even set aside a worry time, a time where you list your worries and think about them, so you don't have to think about them at other times of the day or night.

MINDFULNESS

Mindfulness is an approach to well-being that involves accepting life and living 'in the moment'. This includes paying attention to the present moment and taking time to see what is happening around you in a non judgmental way, rather than focusing on what you are trying to get done and going over your problems again and again. It involves being aware of each thought, feeling or sensation that comes to you and accepting it.

It is not about achieving a particular state or outcome, but more about learning the skills to meet your life the way it is. It tends to involve slowing down a lot to start with as it is difficult to really be present with what is happening right now if you're rushing around. And we do love to get ourselves into that 'rushing' state where we are constantly thinking about what's next. To be truly mindful, you'll notice what is happening with all your sensations at a particular moment.

Why not give it a little try now? Take a deep breath; notice your breath. Is it warm or cool? Does it go in one nostril more than the other? Notice how you feel once you release that breath. Notice what you are sitting on and how that feels. Notice what you can smell, what you can hear, and even what taste is in your mouth. Is that coffee from earlier today still lingering on your taste buds? How do you feel now? Less anxious? Did you worry about anything while doing that exercise? You should find that by doing that one tiny exercise, you will feel much more relaxed. If you can do it every now and then, you'll have started on the journey to a more mindful life.

Mindfulness-based stress reduction (MBSR) is a technique you can learn by following a programme with a therapist or with a computer programme. It is based on meditation techniques, and 'moment-to-moment' awareness – being conscious of what is happening and how you are feeling right now. It is not specific to any specific condition, but can be helpful in coping with many situations.

Mindfulness-based cognitive therapy (MBCT) uses similar techniques to MBSR, but also includes things such as identifying negative thoughts which contribute to conditions like depression, and consciously challenging them. Both these techniques are often used by psychologists, who can help you to work through the process.

PHYSICAL ACTIVITY

Physical activity – completed in moderation – is important for reducing stress levels and preventing some of its damaging effects on the body. Exercise helps to use up the hormones that the body produces under stress and relaxes the muscles. It will also help to strengthen the heart and improve blood circulation. Physical activity also stimulates the body to release endorphins – natural brain chemicals that give you a sense of well-being – and can also help to raise self-esteem and reduce anxiety and depression.

Exercise does not need to be sporty or competitive; you can benefit simply by becoming more active as part of your daily routine. Walking or cycling rather than taking the car or bus, or climbing the stairs rather than using the lift. These small changes can help a lot.

HEALTHY EATING

When things get too hectic or difficult, and you feel under stress, it's often easy to forget about eating well. But what you eat and when you eat can make a big difference to how you feel and how well you cope. It's important to make time for regular food or snacks and not to miss out on meals, such as breakfast. Try not to rush; take time to enjoy what you're eating.

The key to a healthy diet is a variety of different types of food, with a balance of protein, carbohydrate, oily fat and fibre, including plenty of fruit and vegetables. When you are tired and stressed you may feel like a quick sugar rush, but this will leave you feeling tired again later. It's important to keep a steady blood sugar level. Usually we are only aware of this if it has dropped and we suddenly feel weak and hungry; but it may also affect your mood, making you depressed or bad-tempered. If you can, try to eat things that are digested more slowly and give you a steady supply of energy. It's also important to drink plenty of fluids; however, many sweet fizzy drinks and caffeinated drinks can make you feel quite jittery – especially if you are already stressed.

ALTERNATIVE OPTIONS

Alternative and complementary medicine offer a host of alternatives that help to address stress, such things as massage or aromatherapy. Meditation is also helpful in relieving stress and promoting relaxation.

HAVING FUN

Making time for regular leisure activities can help you release tension and to take your mind off the worries of the day. Whether you unwind by soaking in a hot bath, browsing through your favourite books, listening to music, gardening or photography, the important point is to enjoy the activity purely for itself, and to take the focus away from whatever is causing you stress.

I just want to make a personal note here as I'm a bit of a workaholic and tend to prioritise work above all else. In order to get more fun in my life, I've had to make this my top priority, knowing that I'll still do plenty of work as that's just my nature. You may want to consider this for yourself if you too are a workaholic.

DEVELOPING HEALTHY RELATIONSHIPS

Although taking time for yourself to relax is an important way to reduce stress, it is also important to cultivate relationships with other people and spend time socialising with them. Poor relationships and isolation can contribute to burnout, but positive relationships can help to prevent or reduce its onset.

Nurture your closest relationships, such as those with your partner, children or friends. These relationships can help restore energy and alleviate some of the psychological effects of stress, such as feelings of being under-appreciated. Try to put aside what is stressing you out and make sure that the time you spend with loved ones is positive and enjoyable.

Develop casual social relationships, both at work and outside of work. For example, a group from work may decide to go out for a bite to eat. Join them, as this is a great way to see your work colleagues in a different light and to hear about their personal lives rather than discussing work tasks.

Connect with a cause or community group that is personally meaningful to you. Joining a religious, social, or support group can give you a place to talk to like-minded people about how to deal with daily stressors, and can be a way to make new friends. If your line of work has a professional association, you can attend meetings and interact with others coping with the same workplace demands.

Practice healthy communication. Express your feelings to others who will listen, understand, and not judge. Stress and burnout often arise as we are keeping feelings and thoughts inside us, and it can be helpful to let your emotions out in healthy, productive ways.

SELF-ESTEEM

Work on building up your self-esteem. It is helpful and important to have a positive view of ourselves. Some of us have had upbringings we were constantly 'not enough' or 'not good enough', and sadly these feelings often follow us into adulthood. Now is a good time to let those feelings go. Write up a list of achievements (things you are proud of) that you can review when are you feeling stressed and that help to remind you that you are a person of worth. If you do feel that you have some long-term negative beliefs about yourself, you can get schema therapy from a psychologist to help you to shift some of those beliefs.

Make sure you focus on your positives and look after yourself. And by the way, looking after yourself is not being selfish. You may find unhelpful friends or family members tell you you're selfish, or they will say you're selfish to guilt you into doing what they want. What is most important is to make sure you are taking care of yourself. You can't help others if you are not in a good healthy space yourself.

SUMMARY

In summary, to prevent or recover from stress, anxiety or burnout, learn to cultivate methods of personal renewal, self-awareness, and connection with others. Don't be afraid to acknowledge your own needs and find ways to get them met.

6

ADDITIONAL TOOLS

I wanted to include a few other tools and tips, but also didn't want to create too much more reading work for you. So, what follows are a few exercises and tip sheets you may find useful.

Personal Stressor Checklist

Circle all areas of activity or involvement currently present in your life:

Main employment (subdivide roles within your job)
    Other paid work
    Voluntary work
    Main partnership/marriage
    Children
    Parents
    Extended family
    Household maintenance
    Home duties

Study
Personal Finance
Personal health
Others health and well-being
Recreation (self)
Recreation (family)
Personal self-improvement
Education
Pets
Friends and social life
Garden
Home improvement
Other (specify)

- Draw an asterisk next to any life area in which the demands on you have increased recently or there has been anxiety, conflict or strain.
- Draw an asterisk against any area where your supports have been reduced recently.
- Draw an asterisk against any life area that has recently been subject to significant change.
- Draw an asterisk against any life area that is made worse for you by pressure you tend to put on yourself *or* another person tends to put on you.

Note the number of asterisks against each area.

Mark with a tick any life area where things are going well or becoming easier.

For areas asterisked, note the various stressors and write down what could be done, however slight, to reduce each demand or strain factor. Remember that stress is cumulative, so improvements can be made in several areas with cumulative effect. Any small step in the right direction is a good step; even temporary measures can be helpful.

Finally, write down anything that has in the past proved calming, cheering, replenishing or supportive, for example, certain activities, people, places, strategies, books.

Quick Coping Checklist

Find out what triggers your stress – you can then think about what you can stop doing or change to be able to manage the triggers better.

Sort out your worries. Divide them into those you can do something about and those you can't. There are some great little apps that can help you manage your worries – one I know of is called ReachOut Worry Time.

Get organised. Make a list of jobs; tackle one task at a time, alternate dull tasks with interesting ones or schedule fun breaks while doing dull tasks. Aim to do less rather than more. You'll enjoy each task more when you allow enough time to do it, and you may be surprised how much more you can achieve when you slow down a little.

Take control. Get started by doing one task that you can feel you can manage.

Take a regular break. Give yourself a break when you feel that things are becoming overwhelming or they are starting to make you feel stressed. Get a hot drink or a glass of water, or go for a brief walk.

List your achievements. When you've done something you are proud of, write it down. Remember to include the everyday tasks like preparing a meal that you haven't tried before. When you start feeling stressed, read your list and it will give you a boost.

Be active. Physical activity can help you feel calmer, stronger, and better able to deal with emotional stresses. Try to do something you enjoy, for example, take the dog for a walk, dancing, playing a sport, or gardening.

Get a different perspective. Discussing your problems with someone else can help you get new ideas about ways of dealing with your problems. Sharing your thoughts can also help you feel calmer and listened to.

JOIN MY VIP CLUB

Building a relationship with my readers is the best thing about writing. I occasionally send out newsletters with information on upcoming books, recommended books to read, life improvement tools, and great daily rituals.

If you sign up to the mailing list I'll send you my first book *Simplify Your Life* for FREE.

Click here to join my VIP Club

PLEASE LEAVE A REVIEW

Enjoy this book? You can make a big difference.

Reviews are the most powerful tools I have when it comes to getting attention for my books. Much as I'd like to, I don't have the financial muscle of a New York publisher. I can't take out full-page ads in the newspaper or put posters on the subway.

(Not yet, anyway.)

But I do have something much more powerful and effective than that, and it's something those publishers would kill to get their hands on.

A committed and loyal bunch of readers.

Honest reviews of my books help bring them to the attention of other readers.

If you've enjoyed this book I would be very grateful if you could spend just five minutes leaving a review (it can be as short as you like) on the book's Amazon page. You can jump right to the page by clicking below.

AMAZON US
   AMAZON UK
   AMAZON AU

Thank you very much.

ABOUT THE AUTHOR

Sarah has extensive experience in leadership, people manage-ment, mediation, and working with change. She is also the author of *Simplify Your Life* and *Ready For A Career Change*. Sarah's online home is www.sarahoflaherty.com. You can connect with Sarah on Twitter at @sarahof, and on Facebook at www.facebook.com/sarahoflahertymind and you can send her an email at sarah@sarahoflaherty.com if you ever feel so inclined.

.

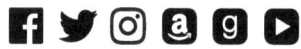

ALSO BY SARAH O'FLAHERTY

Simplify Your Life

Do you wish life was a little easier? Discover the secrets to a simpler, more satisfying life.

Is your life lacking purpose? Are you often stressed and overwhelmed? If so, then it's time for a crash course in the skills that will lead to a more meaningful life. Let successful businesswoman, coach, and author Sarah O'Flaherty be your guide.

Developed from the integration of hundreds of books, a multitude of personal development training formats, and a twenty-year career motivating people, Sarah has created a simple, yet effective, four-part process that will provide you with the skills and confidence you'll need for a happier life.

Each section is presented in a simple style, with tips and easy-to-adopt strategies that will teach you how to unlock your potential. And the best part is, you'll enjoy reading it!

Inside Simplify Your Life you'll discover:

* How to identify your values, strengths, and passions for greater self-awareness and increased life satisfaction.

* How to develop strong healthy relationships so you can benefit from your interactions.

* How to find your purpose or calling for a more meaningful life.

* How to un-complicate your life with some essential tools such as mindfulness.

* And much, much more!

Simplify Your Life is packed with straightforward, honest, and practical advice. If you enjoy easy reads that really add value to your life, then you'll love this book. Sarah takes you straight to the foundational aspects of life that, if you get right, will ensure a satisfying and meaningful life.

Unlock your true potential with Sarah's easy-to-follow guide today!

Click here to purchase

Ready For A Career Change

Feeling trapped in a job you don't like? Discover how to transition into a new career with learnings from people who've done it.

Working long hours, with no satisfaction? Want to start your own business, but not sure you can? Changing careers or setting up your own business isn't easy. Let experienced career coach Sarah O'Flaherty show you how others have made the transition.

Sarah O'Flaherty has a successful business assisting people to improve their life satisfaction and to work through career-transition. After a twenty-year career in advertising, Sarah is now training to become a Clinical Psychologist. Using her own experience and interviews with others who have made major career changes or established their own businesses, Sarah has created nine landmark questions to get you through a career change in one piece. By answering these questions, you'll ensure a transition with minimal stress, while maintaining your relationships, your home, and your sanity.

Inside Ready for a Career Change? you'll discover:

• How to break down the barriers we face when changing jobs so you can make the best decision for you.

• How others have changed careers and their key learnings so you can save time and benefit from their experience.

• The important questions to consider in a career change so you don't waste your time and energy on something that's not right for you.

• The benefits of a career change, such as increased energy and job satisfaction.

• And much, much more!

Ready for a Career Change? Is packed with straightforward, honest, and practical advice that can be your wake-up call to the life that awaits you in a new career. If you like easy reads that tell it to you straight, then you'll love having Sarah on your team.

Buy Ready for a Career Change? to help you make the move to an exciting new life today!

Click here to purchase on Amazon

Click here to purchase with other distributors

Many thanks to all those who assisted me in the process of getting this book produced, including:

Shannon Kuzmich, LaVerne Clark, David Klawitter, Rhonda McGee

Fresh Start, Sarah O'Flaherty. — 1st ed.

❋ Created with Vellum

REFERENCES

1. Fink, G., *Stress Concepts and Cognition, Emotion, and Behaviour.* 2016, Amsterdam: Academic Press.

2. Towers Watson, *The business value of a healthy workforce: A global perspective.* 2014, Towers Watson.

3. Fink, G., *Stress: Definition and history.* Stress science: Neuroendocrinology, 2010: p. 3-9.

4. Kim, J.J. and D.M. Diamond, *The stressed hippocampus, synaptic plasticity and lost memories.* Nat Rev Neuroscience, 2002. 3(6): p. 453-462.

5. Darton, K., *How to manage stress*, Mind, Editor. 2012: London, UK.

6. Parihar, V.K., et al., *Predictable chronic mild stress improves mood, hippocampal neurogenesis and memory.* Molecular Psychiatry, 2011. 16(2): p. 171-183.

7. Hammen, C., *Generation of stress in the course of unipolar depression.* Journal of abnormal psychology (1965), 1991. **100**(4): p. 555-561.

8. Maslach, C., W. Schaufeli, and M. Leiter, *Job burnout.* Annual Review of Psychology, 2001. **52**(1): p. 397-422.

9. Folkman, S. and R.S. Lazarus, *The relationship between coping and emotion: Implications for theory and research.* Social science & medicine, 1988. **26**(3): p. 309-317.

10. Folkman, S., et al., *Dynamics of a stressful encounter: Cognitive appraisal, coping, and encounter outcomes.* Journal of Personality and Social Psychology, 1986. **50**(5): p. 992-1003.

11. Heinonen, K., K. Räikkönen, and L. Keltikangas-Järvinen, *Dispositional optimism: Development over 21 years from the perspectives of perceived temperament and mothering.* Personality and Individual Differences, 2005. **38**(2): p. 425-435.

12339342R00037

Printed in Great Britain
by Amazon